This Journal
Belongs To:

_____

Dedication

This Fitness Planner is dedicated to all the fitness enthusiasts out there who want to be the best version of themselves and document their findings in the process.

You are my inspiration for producing books and I'm honored to be a part of keeping all of your fitness notes and records organized. This journal notebook will help you record the details of your fitness adventures.

Thoughtfully put together with these sections to record: Weekly Progress Tracker, Personal Goals, Weekly Meal Planner, Workout Routine, Daily Meal Tracker, & Notes.

How to Use this Book

The purpose of this book is to keep all of your Fitness notes all in one place. It will help keep you organized.

This Fitness Planner will allow you to accurately document every detail about your fitness adventures.

Here are examples of the prompts for you to fill in and write about your experience in this book:

1. Weekly Progress Tracker - Each week you can record weight, and measurements for left arm, right arm, chest, waist, hips, left thigh, right thigh,

2. Personal Goals - Write your personal goals for the week.

3. Weekly Meal Planner - Plan your menu for the week.

4. Workout Routine Tracker - Log the date, activity, time, sets, distance, reps, weight used, calories burned, water intake, and space to write out your workout routine.

5. Daily Meal Tracker - Record your meals for the day including the date, what you had for breakfast, lunch, dinner, and snacks.

6. Notes - Blank lined space for tracking any important information you want such as your training, if you're doing keto, intermittent fasting, how many calories, eating habits, blood glucose levels, went to the gym, anything you need to work on, grocery list for meal planning etc.

Progress Tracker

Chest

Arm

Waist

Hips

Thigh

WEIGHT:

LEFT ARM:

RIGHT ARM:

CHEST:

WAIST:

HIPS:

LEFT THIGH:

RIGHT THIGH:

My Journey

PERSONAL GOALS:

Meal Planner

MONDAY	NOTES

TUESDAY	NOTES

WEDNESDAY	NOTES

THURSDAY	NOTES

FRIDAY	NOTES

Meal Planner

SATURDAY

NOTES

SUNDAY

NOTES

MY PROGRESS:

My Workout Routine

DATE:

ACTIVITY:

TIME:

DISTANCE:

SETS:

REPS:

WEIGHT USED:

CALORIES BURNED:

WATER INTAKE:

My Routine

Progress Tracker

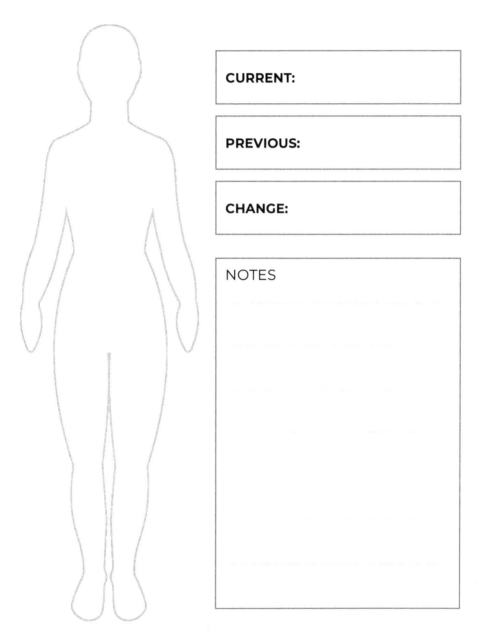

CURRENT:

PREVIOUS:

CHANGE:

NOTES

One day at a time...

Meal Planner

DATE:

BREAKFAST:

_____

_____

LUNCH:

_____

_____

DINNER:

_____

_____

SNACKS:

_____

_____

_____

Progress Tracker

DATE:

	MEASUREMENT:	LOSS/GAIN:
WEIGHT:		
LEFT ARM:		
RIGHT ARM:		
CHEST:		
WAIST:		
HIPS:		
LEFT THIGH:		
RIGHT THIGH:		

Weekly Goals

Meal Planner

	BREAKFAST	LUNCH	DINNER
MON			
TUES			
WED			
THU			
FRI			
SAT			
SUN			

Progress Tracker

Chest

Arm

Waist

Hips

Thigh

STARTING MEASUREMENTS:

WEIGHT:

LEFT ARM:

RIGHT ARM:

CHEST:

WAIST:

HIPS:

LEFT THIGH:

RIGHT THIGH:

My Journey

PERSONAL GOALS:

Meal Planner

MONDAY

NOTES

TUESDAY

NOTES

WEDNESDAY

NOTES

THURSDAY

NOTES

FRIDAY

NOTES

Meal Planner

SATURDAY

NOTES

SUNDAY

NOTES

MY PROGRESS:

My Workout Routine

DATE:

ACTIVITY:

TIME:

DISTANCE:

SETS:

REPS:

WEIGHT USED:

CALORIES BURNED:

WATER INTAKE:

My Routine

Progress Tracker

CURRENT:

PREVIOUS:

CHANGE:

NOTES

One day at a time...

Meal Planner

DATE:

BREAKFAST:

_____

_____

_____

LUNCH:

_____

_____

_____

DINNER:

_____

_____

_____

SNACKS:

_____

_____

_____

_____

Progress Tracker

DATE:

	MEASUREMENT:	LOSS/GAIN:
WEIGHT:		
LEFT ARM:		
RIGHT ARM:		
CHEST:		
WAIST:		
HIPS:		
LEFT THIGH:		
RIGHT THIGH:		

Weekly Goals

Meal Planner

	BREAKFAST	LUNCH	DINNER
MON			
TUES			
WED			
THU			
FRI			
SAT			
SUN			

Progress Tracker

Chest

Arm

Waist

Hips

Thigh

STARTING MEASUREMENTS:

WEIGHT:

LEFT ARM:

RIGHT ARM:

CHEST:

WAIST:

HIPS:

LEFT THIGH:

RIGHT THIGH:

My Journey

PERSONAL GOALS:

Meal Planner

MONDAY

NOTES

TUESDAY

NOTES

WEDNESDAY

NOTES

THURSDAY

NOTES

FRIDAY

NOTES

Meal Planner

SATURDAY

NOTES

SUNDAY

NOTES

MY PROGRESS:

My Workout Routine

DATE:

ACTIVITY:

TIME:

DISTANCE:

SETS:

REPS:

WEIGHT USED:

CALORIES BURNED:

WATER INTAKE:

My Routine

Progress Tracker

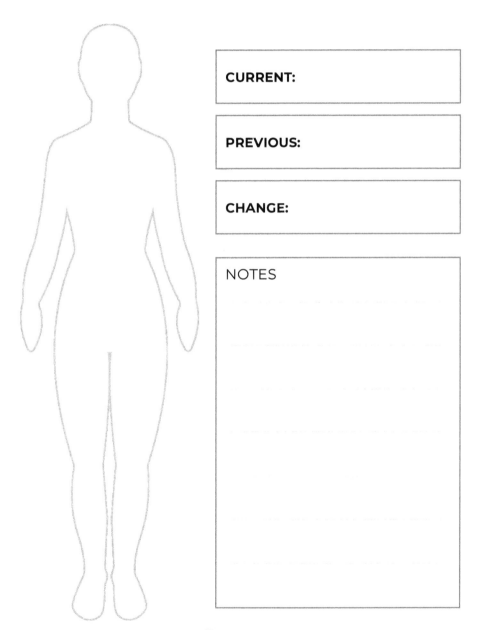

CURRENT:

PREVIOUS:

CHANGE:

NOTES

One day at a time…

Meal Planner

DATE:

BREAKFAST:

_____
_____

LUNCH:

_____
_____

DINNER:

_____
_____

SNACKS:

_____
_____
_____
_____

Progress Tracker

DATE:

	MEASUREMENT:	LOSS/GAIN:
WEIGHT:		
LEFT ARM:		
RIGHT ARM:		
CHEST:		
WAIST:		
HIPS:		
LEFT THIGH:		
RIGHT THIGH:		

Weekly Goals

Meal Planner

	BREAKFAST	LUNCH	DINNER
MON			
TUES			
WED			
THU			
FRI			
SAT			
SUN			

Progress Tracker

Chest

Arm

Waist

Hips

Thigh

WEIGHT:

LEFT ARM:

RIGHT ARM:

CHEST:

WAIST:

HIPS:

LEFT THIGH:

RIGHT THIGH:

My Journey

PERSONAL GOALS:

Meal Planner

MONDAY

NOTES

TUESDAY

NOTES

WEDNESDAY

NOTES

THURSDAY

NOTES

FRIDAY

NOTES

Meal Planner

SATURDAY

NOTES

SUNDAY

NOTES

MY PROGRESS:

My Workout Routine

DATE:

ACTIVITY:

TIME:

DISTANCE:

SETS:

REPS:

WEIGHT USED:

CALORIES BURNED:

WATER INTAKE:

My Routine

Progress Tracker

CURRENT:

PREVIOUS:

CHANGE:

NOTES

One day at a time...

Meal Planner

DATE:

BREAKFAST:

LUNCH:

DINNER:

SNACKS:

Progress Tracker

DATE:

	MEASUREMENT:	LOSS/GAIN:
WEIGHT:		
LEFT ARM:		
RIGHT ARM:		
CHEST:		
WAIST:		
HIPS:		
LEFT THIGH:		
RIGHT THIGH:		

Weekly Goals

Meal Planner

	BREAKFAST	LUNCH	DINNER
MON			
TUES			
WED			
THU			
FRI			
SAT			
SUN			

Progress Tracker

Chest

Arm

Waist

Hips

Thigh

STARTING MEASUREMENTS:

WEIGHT:	
LEFT ARM:	
RIGHT ARM:	
CHEST:	
WAIST:	
HIPS:	
LEFT THIGH:	
RIGHT THIGH:	

My Journey

PERSONAL GOALS:

Meal Planner

MONDAY

NOTES

TUESDAY

NOTES

WEDNESDAY

NOTES

THURSDAY

NOTES

FRIDAY

NOTES

Meal Planner

SATURDAY

NOTES

SUNDAY

NOTES

MY PROGRESS:

My Workout Routine

DATE:

ACTIVITY:

TIME:

DISTANCE:

SETS:

REPS:

WEIGHT USED:

CALORIES BURNED:

WATER INTAKE:

My Routine

Progress Tracker

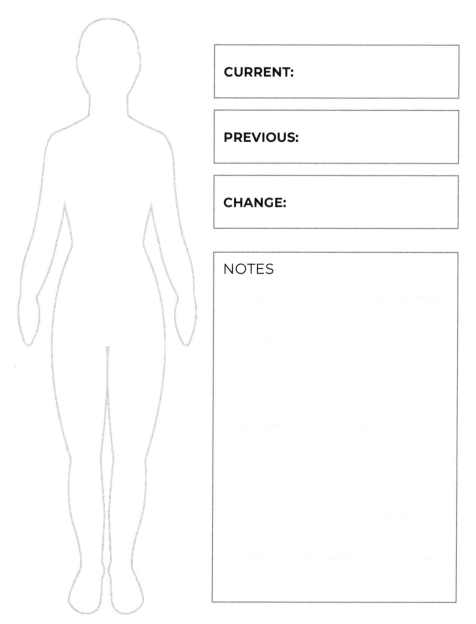

CURRENT:

PREVIOUS:

CHANGE:

NOTES

One day at a time...

Meal Planner

DATE:

BREAKFAST:

_____

_____

_____

LUNCH:

_____

_____

_____

DINNER:

_____

_____

_____

SNACKS:

_____

_____

_____

_____

Progress Tracker

DATE:

	MEASUREMENT:	LOSS/GAIN:
WEIGHT:		
LEFT ARM:		
RIGHT ARM:		
CHEST:		
WAIST:		
HIPS:		
LEFT THIGH:		
RIGHT THIGH:		

Weekly Goals

Meal Planner

	BREAKFAST	LUNCH	DINNER
MON			
TUES			
WED			
THU			
FRI			
SAT			
SUN			

Progress Tracker

Chest

Arm

Waist

Hips

Thigh

STARTING MEASUREMENTS:

WEIGHT:

LEFT ARM:

RIGHT ARM:

CHEST:

WAIST:

HIPS:

LEFT THIGH:

RIGHT THIGH:

My Journey

PERSONAL GOALS:

Meal Planner

MONDAY

NOTES

TUESDAY

NOTES

WEDNESDAY

NOTES

THURSDAY

NOTES

FRIDAY

NOTES

Meal Planner

SATURDAY

NOTES

SUNDAY

NOTES

MY PROGRESS:

My Workout Routine

DATE:

ACTIVITY:

TIME:

DISTANCE:

SETS:

REPS:

WEIGHT USED:

CALORIES BURNED:

WATER INTAKE:

My Routine

Progress Tracker

CURRENT:

PREVIOUS:

CHANGE:

NOTES

One day at a time...

Meal Planner

DATE:

BREAKFAST:

LUNCH:

DINNER:

SNACKS:

Progress Tracker

DATE:

	MEASUREMENT:	LOSS/GAIN:
WEIGHT:		
LEFT ARM:		
RIGHT ARM:		
CHEST:		
WAIST:		
HIPS:		
LEFT THIGH:		
RIGHT THIGH:		

Weekly Goals

Meal Planner

	BREAKFAST	LUNCH	DINNER
MON			
TUES			
WED			
THU			
FRI			
SAT			
SUN			

Progress Tracker

Chest

Arm

Waist

Hips

Thigh

WEIGHT:

LEFT ARM:

RIGHT ARM:

CHEST:

WAIST:

HIPS:

LEFT THIGH:

RIGHT THIGH:

My Journey

PERSONAL GOALS:

Meal Planner

MONDAY

NOTES

TUESDAY

NOTES

WEDNESDAY

NOTES

THURSDAY

NOTES

FRIDAY

NOTES

Meal Planner

SATURDAY

NOTES

SUNDAY

NOTES

MY PROGRESS:

My Workout Routine

DATE:

ACTIVITY:

TIME:

DISTANCE:

SETS:

REPS:

WEIGHT USED:

CALORIES BURNED:

WATER INTAKE:

My Routine

Progress Tracker

CURRENT:

PREVIOUS:

CHANGE:

NOTES

One day at a time…

Meal Planner

DATE:

BREAKFAST:

LUNCH:

DINNER:

SNACKS:

Progress Tracker

DATE:

	MEASUREMENT:	LOSS/GAIN:
WEIGHT:		
LEFT ARM:		
RIGHT ARM:		
CHEST:		
WAIST:		
HIPS:		
LEFT THIGH:		
RIGHT THIGH:		

Weekly Goals

Meal Planner

	BREAKFAST	LUNCH	DINNER
MON			
TUES			
WED			
THU			
FRI			
SAT			
SUN			

Progress Tracker

Chest

Arm

Waist

Hips

Thigh

| WEIGHT: |
| LEFT ARM: |
| RIGHT ARM: |
| CHEST: |
| WAIST: |
| HIPS: |
| LEFT THIGH: |
| RIGHT THIGH: |

My Journey

PERSONAL GOALS:

Meal Planner

MONDAY

NOTES

TUESDAY

NOTES

WEDNESDAY

NOTES

THURSDAY

NOTES

FRIDAY

NOTES

Meal Planner

SATURDAY

NOTES

SUNDAY

NOTES

MY PROGRESS:

My Workout Routine

DATE:

ACTIVITY:

TIME:

DISTANCE:

SETS:

REPS:

WEIGHT
USED:

CALORIES
BURNED:

WATER INTAKE:

My Routine

Progress Tracker

CURRENT:

PREVIOUS:

CHANGE:

NOTES

One day at a time...

Meal Planner

DATE:

BREAKFAST:

LUNCH:

DINNER:

SNACKS:

Progress Tracker

DATE:

	MEASUREMENT:	LOSS/GAIN:
WEIGHT:		
LEFT ARM:		
RIGHT ARM:		
CHEST:		
WAIST:		
HIPS:		
LEFT THIGH:		
RIGHT THIGH:		

Weekly Goals

Meal Planner

	BREAKFAST	LUNCH	DINNER
MON			
TUES			
WED			
THU			
FRI			
SAT			
SUN			

Progress Tracker

Chest

Arm

Waist

Hips

Thigh

| WEIGHT: |
| LEFT ARM: |
| RIGHT ARM: |
| CHEST: |
| WAIST: |
| HIPS: |
| LEFT THIGH: |
| RIGHT THIGH: |

My Journey

PERSONAL GOALS:

Meal Planner

MONDAY

NOTES

TUESDAY

NOTES

WEDNESDAY

NOTES

THURSDAY

NOTES

FRIDAY

NOTES

Meal Planner

SATURDAY

NOTES

SUNDAY

NOTES

MY PROGRESS:

My Workout Routine

DATE:

ACTIVITY:

TIME:

DISTANCE:

SETS:

REPS:

WEIGHT USED:

CALORIES BURNED:

WATER INTAKE:

My Routine

Progress Tracker

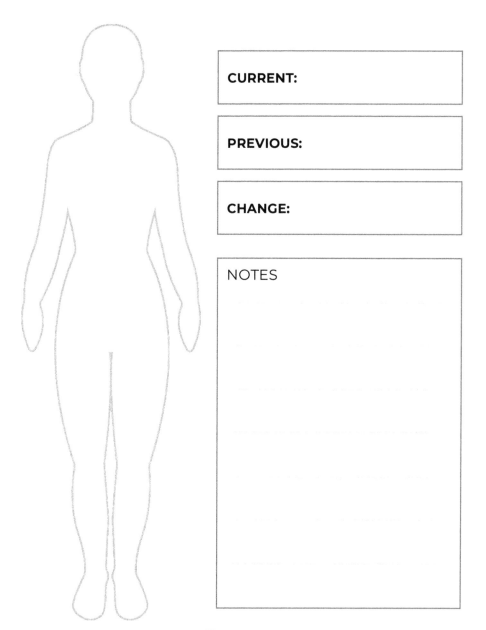

CURRENT:

PREVIOUS:

CHANGE:

NOTES

One day at a time...

Meal Planner

DATE:

BREAKFAST:

LUNCH:

DINNER:

SNACKS:

Progress Tracker

DATE:

	MEASUREMENT:	LOSS/GAIN:
WEIGHT:		
LEFT ARM:		
RIGHT ARM:		
CHEST:		
WAIST:		
HIPS:		
LEFT THIGH:		
RIGHT THIGH:		

Weekly Goals

Meal Planner

	BREAKFAST	LUNCH	DINNER
MON			
TUES			
WED			
THU			
FRI			
SAT			
SUN			

Progress Tracker

Chest

Arm

Waist

Hips

Thigh

STARTING MEASUREMENTS:

WEIGHT:	
LEFT ARM:	
RIGHT ARM:	
CHEST:	
WAIST:	
HIPS:	
LEFT THIGH:	
RIGHT THIGH:	

My Journey

PERSONAL GOALS:

Meal Planner

MONDAY	NOTES

TUESDAY	NOTES

WEDNESDAY	NOTES

THURSDAY	NOTES

FRIDAY	NOTES

Meal Planner

SATURDAY

NOTES

SUNDAY

NOTES

MY PROGRESS:

My Workout Routine

DATE:

ACTIVITY:

TIME:

DISTANCE:

SETS:

REPS:

WEIGHT USED:

CALORIES BURNED:

WATER INTAKE:

My Routine

Progress Tracker

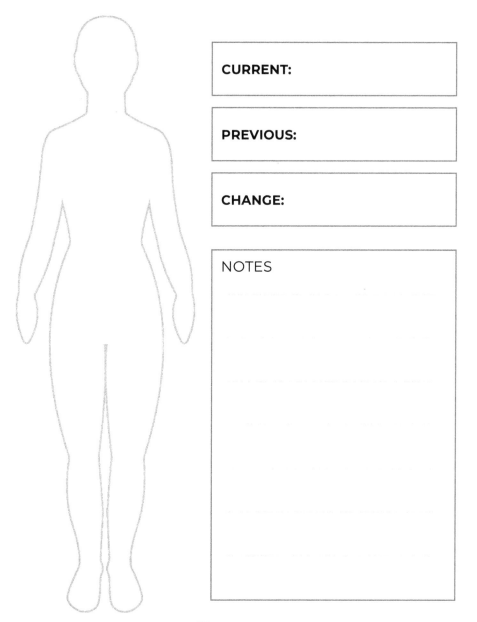

CURRENT:

PREVIOUS:

CHANGE:

NOTES

One day at a time…

Meal Planner

DATE:

BREAKFAST:

LUNCH:

DINNER:

SNACKS:

Progress Tracker

DATE:

	MEASUREMENT:	LOSS/GAIN:
WEIGHT:		
LEFT ARM:		
RIGHT ARM:		
CHEST:		
WAIST:		
HIPS:		
LEFT THIGH:		
RIGHT THIGH:		

Weekly Goals

Meal Planner

	BREAKFAST	LUNCH	DINNER
MON			
TUES			
WED			
THU			
FRI			
SAT			
SUN			

Printed in the USA
CPSIA information can be obtained
at www.ICGtesting.com
LVHW011937271223
767589LV00011B/745